THE RENAL ~~DIET~~

COOKBOOK FOR

BEGINNERS

EASY, FAST AND SIMPLE RECIPES

PERFECT FOR BOOSTING BRAIN

ACTIVITY AND HAS

ANTI-INFLAMMATORY PROPERTIES

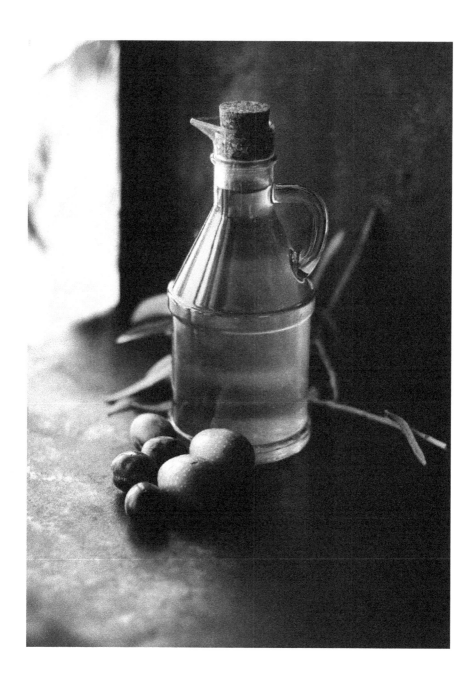

Table of contents

—

As befitting its nature, it is presented without assurance regarding its prolonged validity or interim quality. Trademarks that are mentioned are done without written consent and can in no way be considered an endorsement from the trademark holder.

Turkey Meatballs

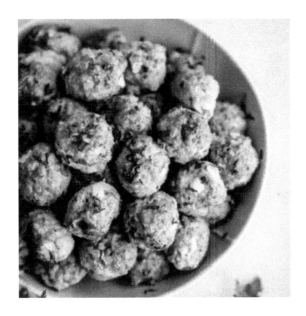

Preparation Time: 10 minutes

Cooking Time: 22 minutes

Servings: 12

Ingredients:

- 1 lb. ground turkey
- 1 large egg
- 1/4 cup bread crumbs
- 2 tablespoons onion, finely chopped
- 1 teaspoon garlic powder
- 1/2 teaspoons black pepper
- 1/4 cup canola oil

- 6 oz. grape jelly
- 1/4 cup chili sauce

Directions:

1. Start by tossing turkey meat along with all other ingredients in a bowl. Stir well until evenly mixed, then roll small meatballs out of this mixture. It will make as many as 48 meatballs.
2. Place these meatballs at the bottom of an Instant Pot. Whisk chili sauce with jelly in a suitable bowl and cook it for 2 minutes in the microwave. Mix well, then add this batter to the meatballs.
3. Cook the saucy meatballs for 20 minutes approximately on Manual Mode at High pressure. Serve immediately.

Nutrition:

Calories 127

Fats 4 g

Sodium 121 mg

Carbs 14 g

Protein 9 g

Phosphorus 0 mg

Potassium 0 mg

VEGETABLE CORN BREAD

Preparation Time: 10 minutes

Cooking Time: 30 minutes

Servings: 6

Ingredients:

- 1 cup almond flour
- 1 cup plain cornmeal
- 1 tablespoon sugar
- 2 teaspoons baking powder
- 1 teaspoon chili powder
- 1/4 teaspoons black pepper
- 1 cup rice milk, unenriched
- 1 egg
- 1 egg white
- 2 tablespoons canola oil
- 1/2 cup scallions, finely chopped
- 1/4 cup carrots, finely grated
- 1 garlic clove, minced

Directions:

1. Now begin mixing the flour with sugar, baking powder, cornmeal, pepper, and chili powder in a suitable mixing bowl. Pour in oil, milk, egg white, and egg. Stir well until it's smooth, then fold in garlic, carrots, and scallions.
2. Mix well evenly, then spread this batter in an 8-inch baking dish, greased with cooking spray. Put a cup of water into the bottom of the Instant Pot.

3. Place a steamer rack in the pot and set the baking dish over it. Cook the corn batter for 30 minutes approximately on Manual mode with High pressure until golden brown. Slice and serve fresh.

Nutrition:

Calories 188

Fats 5 g

Sodium 155 mg

Carbs 31 g

Protein 5 g

Phosphorus 98.6 mg

Potassium 138.6 mg

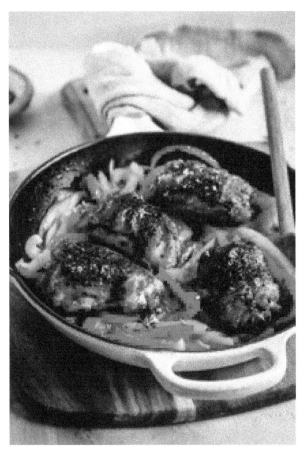

Preparation Time: 10 minutes

Cooking Time: 15 minutes

Servings: 6

Ingredients:

- 1 medium onion, chopped
- 12 fresh jalapenos peppers
- 12 fresh banana peppers
- 2 lbs. boneless, skinless chicken breast

Directions:

1. Slice the onion in quarters. Grease the rack of the instant with cooking spray. Discard the pepper's seed and chop them in half lengthwise.
2. Cut the chicken into 24 pieces, divide them into the peppers, and then top the chicken with an onion slice. Put a cup of water inside your Instant Pot.
3. Place the rack in the pot and arrange the peppers in the frame. Seal the lid and select the manual mode with high pressure for 15 minutes. Serve the peppers.

Nutrition:

Calories 115

Fats 7 g

Sodium 156 mg

Carbs 11 g

Protein 2 g

Potassium 556 mg

Phosphorus 146 mg

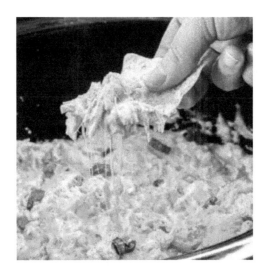

Preparation Time: 10 minutes

Cooking Time: 7 minutes

Servings: 4

Ingredients:

- 4 ounces' cream cheese
- 1/2 cup bottled roasted red peppers
- 1 cup reduced-fat sour cream
- 4 teaspoons hot pepper sauce
- 2 cups cooked, shredded chicken

Directions:

1. Blend ½ cup of drained red peppers in a food processor until smooth. Now evenly mix cream cheese, sour cream, and 2 tablespoons Tabasco sauce with the bowl's peppers.

2. Toss in chicken; hot sauce, then transfers the mixture to the Instant Pot. Cook on high within 7 minutes. Serve.

Nutrition:

Calories 73

Fats 5 g

Sodium 66 mg

Carbs 2 g

Protein 5 g

Potassium 161 mg

Phosphorus 236 mg

PROSCIUTTO-WRAPPED ASPARAGUS

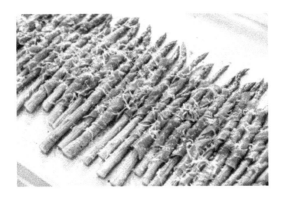

Preparation Time: 10 minutes

Cooking Time: 3 minutes

Servings: 4

Ingredients:

- 1lb thick Asparagus
- 8oz thinly sliced Prosciutto
- Black pepper to taste

Directions:

1. Put 1 cup of water inside your pot and place a rack over it. Take an asparagus spear and wrap it with a prosciutto slice.
2. Continue wrapping all the asparagus spears this way. Place the spears over the rack and then seal the lid.
3. Cook for 3 minutes on Manual mode at High pressure. Serve wrapped spears with black pepper on top. Enjoy.

Nutrition:

Calories 71

Fats 3 g

Sodium 96 mg

Carbs 1 g

Protein 10 g

Potassium 129 mg

Phosphorus 82.4 mg

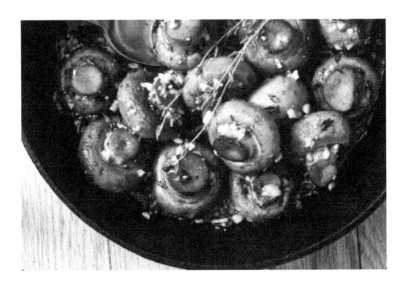

Preparation Time: 10 minutes

Cooking Time: 20 minutes

Servings: 4

Ingredients:

- 2 tablespoons olive oil
- 1 lb. small button mushrooms
- 2 tablespoons butter
- 2 teaspoons minced garlic
- 1/2 teaspoons fresh thyme

Directions:

1. Start by preheating the Instant pot on Sauté mode. Add olive oil and mushrooms to the pool and sauté for 5 minutes.

2. Add garlic, thyme, and butter, then mix well to coat. Seal the pot's lid and cook for 15 minutes on Manual mode with high pressure. Serve.

Nutrition:

Calories 118

Fats 7 g

Sodium 166 mg

Carbs 12 g

Protein 2 g

Potassium 395.1 mg

Phosphorus 98 mg

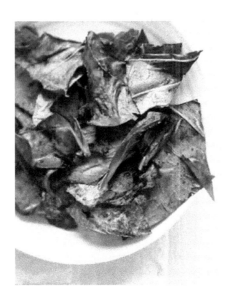

Preparation Time: 5 minutes

Cooking Time: 20 minutes

Servings: 4

Ingredients:

- 1 bunch of collard greens
- 1 teaspoon of extra-virgin olive oil
- Juice of ½ lemon
- ½ teaspoon of garlic powder
- ¼ teaspoon of freshly ground black pepper

Directions:

1. Preheat the oven to 350°F. Line a baking sheet with parchment paper. Cut the collards into 2-by-2-inch squares and pat dry with paper towels.
2. Toss greens with the olive oil, lemon juice, garlic powder, and pepper in a large bowl. Put the dressing into the gardens, then massage using your hands until evenly coated.
3. Arrange the collards in a single layer on the baking sheet, and cook for 8 minutes. Flip and cook again within 8 minutes, until crisp. Remove from oven, let cool.

Nutrition:

Calories: 24

Fat: 1g

Carbohydrates: 3g

Protein: 1g

Phosphorus: 6mg

Potassium: 72mg

Sodium: 8mg

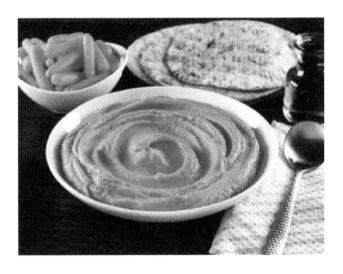

Preparation Time: 10 minutes

Cooking Time: 10 minutes

Servings: 8

Ingredients:

- 1 red bell pepper
- 1 can of chickpeas, drained
- Juice of 1 lemon
- 2 tablespoons of tahini
- 2 garlic cloves
- 2 tablespoons of extra-virgin olive oil

Directions:

1. Move the rack of the oven to the highest position. Heat the broiler to high. Core the pepper and cut it into three or four large pieces. Arrange them on a baking sheet, skin-side up.
2. Broil the peppers for 5 to 10 minutes, until the skins are charred. Remove from the oven, then transfer the peppers to a small bowl. Cover with plastic wrap and let them steam for 10 to 15 minutes, until cool enough to handle.
3. Peel the burnt skin off the peppers, and place the peppers in a blender. Add the chickpeas, lemon juice, tahini, garlic, and olive oil. Wait until smooth, then add up to 1 tablespoon of water to adjust consistency as desired.

Nutrition:

Calories: 103

Fat: 6g

Carbohydrates: 10g

Protein: 3g

Phosphorus: 58mg

Potassium: 91mg

Sodium: 72mg

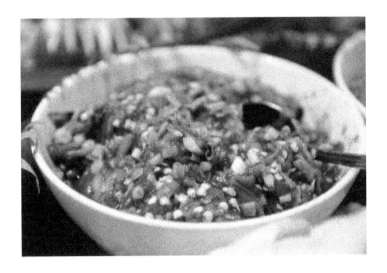

Preparation Time: 10 minutes

Cooking Time: 30 minutes

Servings: 4

Ingredients:

- 1 pound of Thai eggplant (or Japanese or Chinese eggplant)
- 2 tablespoons of rice vinegar
- 2 teaspoons of sugar
- 1 teaspoon of low-sodium soy sauce
- 1 jalapeño pepper
- 2 garlic cloves
- ¼ cup of chopped basil
- Cut vegetables or crackers for serving

Directions:

1. Preheat the oven to 425°F to get it ready. Pierce every eggplant with a skewer or knife. Put on a rimmed baking sheet and cook within 30 minutes. Let cool, cut in half, and scoop out the flesh of the eggplant into a blender.
2. Add the rice vinegar, sugar, soy sauce, jalapeño, garlic, and basil to the blender. Process until smooth. Serve with cut vegetables or crackers.

Nutrition:

Calories: 40

Fat: 0g

Carbohydrates: 10g

Protein: 2g

Phosphorus: 34mg

Potassium: 284mg

Sodium: 47mg

Coconut Pancakes

Preparation Time: 5 minutes

Cooking Time: 10 minutes

Servings: 2

Ingredients:

- 2 free-range egg whites
- 2 tbsp of all-purpose white flour
- 3 tbsp of coconut shavings
- 2 tbsp of coconut milk (optional)
- 1 tbsp of coconut oil

Directions:

1. Get a bowl and combine all the ingredients. Mix well until you get a thick batter. Heat a skillet on medium heat and heat the coconut oil.
2. Pour half the mixture to the pan's center, forming a pancake, and cook through for 3-4 minutes on each side. Serve with your choice of berries on the top.

Nutrition:

Calories: 177

Fat: 13g

Carbohydrates: 12g

Phosphorus: 37mg

Potassium: 133mg

Sodium: 133mg

Protein: 5g

SPICED PEACHES

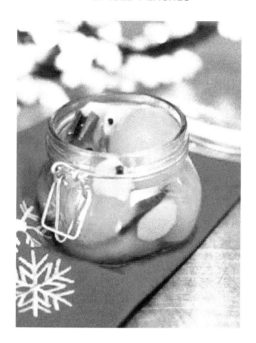

Preparation Time: 5 minutes

Cooking Time: 10 minutes

Servings: 2

Ingredients:

- 1 cup of canned peaches in their juices
- 1/2 tsp of cornstarch
- 1 tsp of ground cloves
- 1 tsp of ground cinnamon
- 1 tsp of ground nutmeg
- 1/2 lemon zest
- 1/2 cup of water

Directions:

1. Drain peaches. Combine water, cornstarch, cinnamon, nutmeg, ground cloves, and lemon zest in a pan on the stove. Heat on medium heat and add peaches. Boil, then adjust the heat and simmer for 10 minutes. Serve warm.

Nutrition:

Calories: 70

Fat: 1g

Carbohydrates: 18g

Phosphorus: 26mg

Potassium: 184mg

Sodium: 9mg

Protein: 1g

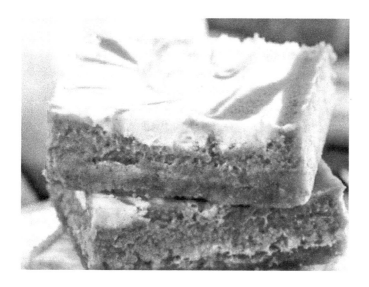

Preparation Time: 10 minutes

Cooking Time: 50 minutes

Servings: 4

Ingredients:

- 2 ½ tbsp of unsalted butter
- 4 oz. of cream cheese
- 1/2 cup of all-purpose white flour
- 3 tbsp of golden-brown sugar
- 1/4 cup of granulated sugar
- 1/2 cup of puréed pumpkin
- 2 egg whites
- 1 tsp of ground cinnamon
- 1 tsp of ground nutmeg
- 1 tsp of vanilla extract

Directions:

1. Set the oven to 350°F. Mix the flour and brown sugar in a mixing bowl. Mix in the butter with your fingertips to form 'breadcrumbs.'
2. Place 3/4 of this mixture into the bottom of an ovenproof dish. Bake in the oven for 15 minutes and remove to cool.
3. Lightly whisk the egg and fold in the cream cheese, sugar (or substitute stevia), pumpkin, cinnamon, nutmeg, and vanilla until smooth.
4. Pour this mixture over the oven-baked base and sprinkle with the rest of the breadcrumbs from earlier. Put it back in the oven, then bake within 30–35 minutes. Allow to cool and slice to serve.

Nutrition:

Calories: 296

Fat: 17g

Carbohydrates: 30g

Phosphorus: 62mg

Potassium: 164g

Sodium: 159mg

Protein: 5g

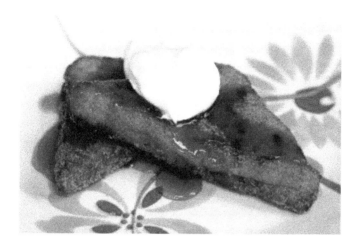

Preparation Time: 10 minutes

Cooking Time: 8 minutes

Servings: 4

Ingredients:

- 4 slices of white bread, cut in half diagonally
- 3 whole eggs and 1 egg white
- 1 cup of plain almond milk
- 2 tbsp of canola oil
- 1 tsp of cinnamon

Directions:

1. Preheat your oven to 400F. Beat the eggs and the almond milk. Heat the oil in a pan. Dip each bread slice/triangle into the egg and almond milk mixture.

2. Fry in the pan, then place the toasts on a baking sheet and cook in the oven for another 5 minutes. Serve warm and drizzle with some honey, icing sugar, or cinnamon on top.

Nutrition:

Calories: 293.75

Carbohydrate: 25.3g

Protein: 9.27g

Sodium: 211g

Potassium: 97mg

Phosphorus: 165mg

Fat: 16.50g

Puff Oven Pancakes

Preparation Time: 5 minutes

Cooking Time: 30 minutes

Servings: 4

Ingredients:

- 2 large eggs
- ½ cup of rice flour
- ½ cup of rice milk
- 2 tbsp. of unsalted butter
- 1/8 tsp of salt

Directions:

1. Preheat the oven to 400°F. Grease a 10-inch skillet or Pyrex with the butter and heat in the oven until it melts.
2. Beat the eggs and whisk in the rice milk, flour and salt in a mixing bowl until smooth. Take off the skillet or pie dish from the oven.
3. Transfer the batter directly into the skillet and put back in the oven for 25–30 minutes. Place in a serving dish and cut into 4 portions. Serve hot with honey or icing sugar on top.

Nutrition:

Calories: 159.75

Carbohydrate: 17g

Protein: 5g

Sodium: 120g

Potassium: 52mg

Phosphorus: 66.25mg

Fat: 9g

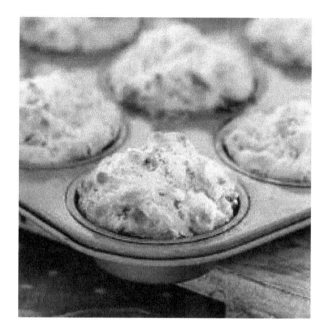

Preparation Time: 5 minutes

Cooking Time: 35 minutes

Servings: 12

Ingredients:

- 2 cups of corn flakes
- ½ cup of unfortified almond milk
- 4 large eggs
- 2 tbsp. of olive oil
- 1/2 cup of almond milk
- 1 medium white onion, sliced
- 1 cup of plain Greek yogurt
- ¼ cup of pecans, chopped

- 1 tbsp of mixed seasoning blend, e.g., Mrs. dash

Directions:

1. Preheat the oven to 350°F. Heat the olive oil in the pan. Sauté the onions with the pecans and seasoning blend for a couple of minutes.
2. Add the rest of the ingredients and toss well. Split the mixture into 12 small muffin cups (lightly greased) and bake for 30–35 minutes or until an inserted knife or toothpick is coming out clean. Serve warm or keep at room temperature for a couple of days.

Nutrition:

Calories: 106.58

Carbohydrate: 8.20g

Protein: 4.77g

Sodium: 51.91mg

Potassium: 87.83 mg

Phosphorus: 49.41 mg

Fat: 5 g

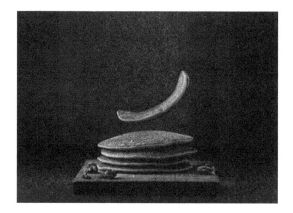

Preparation Time: 5 minutes

Cooking Time: 20 minutes

Servings: 10

Ingredients:

- 2/3 cups of all-purpose flour
- 4 large eggs
- 2 tbsp. of sugar
- ½ tsp. of lemon zest
- 1 cup of low-fat milk
- ¼ tsp. of vanilla extract

Directions:

1. Mix flour and sugar, then whisk in the eggs and combine well in a medium. Put then the milk, vanilla, and lemon zest to the mix and whisk well.

2. Spray a small 8–10-inch pan with cooking spray and pour around 4 tbsp of the mixture and distribute evenly by tilting the pan from one side to another.
3. Cook until the batter or mixture is solid and light golden brown (around 50 seconds on each side). Flip. Repeat the process with the remaining batter.

Nutrition:

Calories: 74

Carbohydrate: 10g

Protein: 4g

Sodium: 39mg

Potassium: 73mg

Phosphorus: 73mg

Fat: 2g

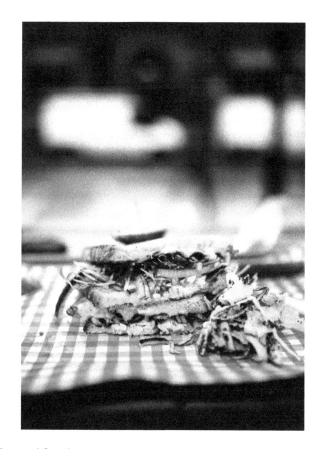

Preparation Time: 10 minutes

Cooking Time: 10 minutes

Servings: 2

Ingredients:

- 2 bowls of cooked chicken
- 1/2 cup of low-fat mayonnaise
- 1/2 cup of green bell pepper
- 1 cup of pieces pineapple

- 1/3 cup of carrots
- 4 slices of flatbread
- 1/2 tsp of black pepper

Directions:

1. Prepare aside the diced chicken and drain pineapple, adding green bell pepper, black pepper, and carrots. Combine all in a bowl and refrigerate until chilled. Later on, serve the chicken salad on the flatbread. Enjoy!

Nutrition:

Calories: 345

Protein: 22g

Carbohydrate: 0g

Sodium: 395mg

Fat: 0g

Potassium: 330mg

Phosphorus: 165mg

Chicken, Charred Tomato, and Broccoli Salad

Preparation Time: 10 minutes

Cooking Time: 30 minutes

Servings: 6

Ingredients:

- ¼ cup of lemon juice
- ½ tsp of chili powder
- 1 ½ lb. of boneless chicken breast
- 1 ½ lb. of a medium tomato
- 1 tsp of freshly ground pepper
- 1 tsp of sea salt
- 4 cups of broccoli florets
- 5 tbsp of extra virgin olive oil, divided into 2 and 3 tablespoons

Directions:

1. Place the chicken in a skillet and add just enough water to cover the chicken. Bring to a simmer over high heat.
2. Reduce the heat once the liquid boils and cook the chicken thoroughly for 12 minutes. Once cooked, shred the chicken into bite-sized pieces.
3. On a large pot, bring water to a boil and add the broccoli. Cook for 5 minutes until slightly tender. Drain and rinse the broccoli using cold water. Set aside.
4. Core the tomatoes and cut them crosswise. Discard the seeds and set the tomatoes cut-side down on paper towels. Pat them dry.

———

5. In a heavy skillet, heat the pan over high heat. Brush the slice sides of the tomatoes with olive oil and place them on the pan. Cook the tomatoes until the sides are charred. Set aside.
6. In the same pan, heat the remaining 3 tablespoon olive oil over medium heat. Stir the salt, chili powder, and pepper and stir for 45 seconds.
7. Pour over the lemon juice and remove the pan from the heat. Plate the broccoli, shredded chicken, and chili powder mixture dressing.

Nutrition:

Calories: 277

Carbs: 6g

Protein: 28g

Fat: 9g

Phosphorus: 292mg

Potassium: 719mg

Sodium: 560mg

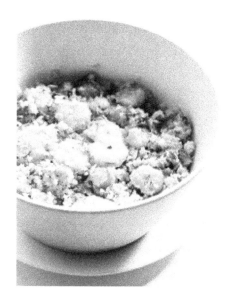

Preparation time: 10 minutes

Cooking time: 10 minutes

Servings: 4

Ingredients:

- 5 cups cauliflower florets
- 3 tablespoons coconut oil
- 4 ginger slices, grated
- 1 tablespoon coconut vinegar
- 3 garlic cloves, minced
- 1 tablespoon chives, minced
- A pinch of sea salt
- Black pepper to taste

Directions:

1. Pulse the cauliflower using your food processor. Heat-up a pan with the oil over medium-high heat, add ginger, stir and cook for 3 minutes.
2. Add cauliflower rice and garlic, stir and cook for 7 minutes. Add salt, black pepper, vinegar, chives, stir, cook for a few seconds more, divide between plates, and serve.

Nutrition:

Calories 125

Fat 10.4g

Carbs 79g

Protein 2.7g

Phosphorus 35 mg

Potassium 228.3 mg

Sodium 21.9 mg

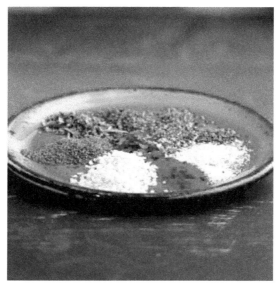

Preparation time: 10 minutes

Cooking time: 0 minutes

Servings: ½ cup

Ingredients:

- ¼ cup celery seed
- 1 tablespoon dried basil
- 1 tablespoon dried oregano
- 1 tablespoon dried thyme
- 1 tablespoon onion powder
- 2 teaspoons garlic powder
- 1 teaspoon freshly ground black pepper
- ½ teaspoon ground cloves

Directions:

1. Mix the celery seed, basil, oregano, thyme, onion powder, garlic powder, pepper, and cloves in a small bowl. Store for up to 1 month.

Nutrition:

Calories: 7

Fat: 0g

Sodium: 2mg

Carbohydrates: 1g

Phosphorus: 9mg

Potassium: 27mg

Protein: 0g

Phosphorus-Free Baking Powder

Preparation time: 5 minutes

Cooking time: 0 minutes

Servings: 1

Ingredients:

- ¾ cup cream of tartar
- ¼ cup baking soda

Directions:

1. Mix the cream of tartar plus baking soda in a small bowl. Sift the mixture together several times to mix thoroughly. Store the baking powder in a sealed container in a cool, dark place for up to 1 month.

Nutrition:

Calories: 6

Fat: 0g

Sodium: 309mg

Carbohydrates: 1g

Phosphorus: 0g

Potassium: 341mg

Protein: 0g

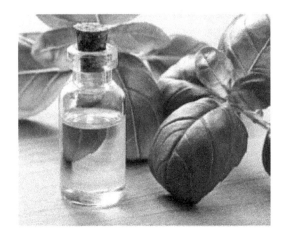

Preparation time: 15 minutes

Cooking time: 4 minutes

Servings: 3

Ingredients:

- 2 cups olive oil
- 2½ cups fresh basil leaves patted dry

Directions:

1. Put the olive oil plus basil leaves in a food processor or blender, and pulse until the leaves are coarsely chopped.
2. Transfer these to a medium saucepan, and place over medium heat. Heat the oil, occasionally stirring, until it just starts to simmer along the edges, about 4 minutes. Remove, then let it stand until cool, about 2 hours.

3. Pour the oil through a fine-mesh sieve or doubled piece of cheesecloth into a container. Store the basil oil in an airtight glass container in the refrigerator for up to 2 months.
4. Before using for dressings, remove the oil from the refrigerator and let it come to room temperature or scoop out cold spoonsful for cooking.

Nutrition:

Calories: 40

Fat: 5g

Sodium: 0g

Carbohydrates: 0g

Phosphorus: 0g

Potassium: 0g

Protein: 0g

Basil Pesto

Preparation time: 15 minutes

Cooking time: 0 minutes

Servings: 1 ½ cups

Ingredients:

- 2 cups gently packed fresh basil leaves
- 2 garlic cloves
- 2 tablespoons pine nuts
- ¼ cup olive oil
- 2 tablespoons freshly squeezed lemon juice

Directions:

1. Pulse the basil, garlic, plus pine nuts using a food processor or blender within about 3 minutes. Drizzle the olive oil into this batter, and pulse until thick paste forms.
2. Put the lemon juice, and pulse until well blended. Store the pesto in a sealed glass container in the refrigerator for up to 2 weeks.

Nutrition:

Calories: 22

Fat: 2g

Sodium: 0mg

Carbohydrates: 0g

Phosphorus: 3mg

Potassium: 10mg

Protein: 0g

LOW-SODIUM MAYONNAISE

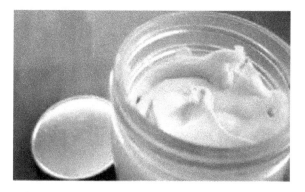

Preparation time: 15 minutes

Cooking time: 0 minutes

Servings: 3

Ingredients:

- 2 egg yolks
- 1 teaspoon Dijon mustard
- 1 teaspoon honey
- 2 tablespoons white vinegar
- 2 tablespoons freshly squeezed lemon juice
- 2 cups olive oil

Directions:

1. Mix the egg yolks, mustard, honey, vinegar, and lemon juice in a large bowl. Mix in the olive oil in a thin stream. You can store this in a glass container in the refrigerator for up to 2 weeks.

Nutrition:

Calories: 83

Fat: 9g

Sodium: 2mg

Carbohydrates: 0g

Phosphorus: 2mg

Potassium: 3mg

Protein: 0g

CITRUS AND MUSTARD MARINADE

Preparation time: 15 minutes

Cooking time: 0 minutes

Servings: ¾ cup

Ingredients:

- ¼ cup freshly squeezed lemon juice
- ¼ cup freshly squeezed orange juice
- ¼ cup Dijon mustard
- 2 tablespoons honey
- 2 teaspoons chopped fresh thyme

Directions:

1. Mix the lemon juice, orange juice, mustard, honey, and thyme until well blended in a medium bowl. Store the marinade in a sealed glass container in the refrigerator for up to 3 days. Shake before using it.

Nutrition:

Calories: 35

Fat: 0g

Sodium: 118mg

Carbohydrates: 8g

Phosphorus: 14mg

Potassium: 52mg

Protein: 1g

Fiery Honey Vinaigrette

Preparation time: 15 minutes

Cooking time: 0 minutes

Servings: ¾ cup

Ingredients:

- 1/3 cup freshly squeezed lime juice
- ¼ cup honey
- ¼ cup olive oil
- 1 teaspoon chopped fresh basil leaves
- ½ teaspoon red pepper flakes

Directions:

1. Mix the lime juice, honey, olive oil, basil, and red pepper flakes in a medium bowl, until well blended. Store the dressing in a glass container, and store it in the fridge for up to 1 week.

Nutrition:

Calories: 125

Fat: 9g

Sodium: 1mg

Carbohydrates: 13g

Phosphorus: 1mg

Potassium: 24mg

Protein: 0g

BUTTERMILK HERB DRESSING

Preparation time: 15 minutes

Cooking time: 0 minutes

Servings: 1 ½ cup

Ingredients:

- ½ cup skim milk
- ½ cup Low-Sodium Mayonnaise
- 2 tablespoons apple cider vinegar
- ½ scallion, green part only, chopped
- 1 tablespoon chopped fresh dill
- 1 teaspoon chopped fresh thyme
- ½ teaspoon minced garlic
- Freshly ground black pepper

Directions:

1. Mix the milk, mayonnaise, and vinegar until smooth in a medium bowl. Whisk in the scallion, dill, thyme, and garlic. Season with pepper. Store.

Nutrition:

Calories: 31

Fat: 2g

Sodium: 19mg

Carbohydrates: 2g

Phosphorus: 13mg

Potassium: 26mg

Poppy Seed Dressing

Preparation time: 15 minutes

Cooking time: 0 minutes

Servings: 2 cups

Ingredients:

- ½ cup apple cider or red wine vinegar
- 1/3 cup honey
- ¼ cup freshly squeezed lemon juice
- 1 tablespoon Dijon mustard
- 1 cup olive oil
- ½ small sweet onion, minced
- 2 tablespoons poppy seeds

Directions:

1. Mix the vinegar, honey, lemon juice, and mustard in a small bowl. Whisk in the oil, onion, and poppy seeds. Store the dressing in a sealed glass container in the refrigerator for up to 2 weeks.

Nutrition:

Calories: 151

Fat: 14g

Sodium: 12mg

Carbohydrates: 7g

Phosphorus: 13mg

Potassium: 30mg

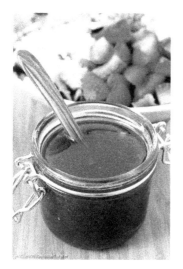

Mediterranean Dressing

Preparation time: 15 minutes

Cooking time: 0 minutes

Servings: 1 cup

Ingredients:

- ½ cup balsamic vinegar
- 1 teaspoon honey
- ½ teaspoon minced garlic
- 1 tablespoon dried parsley
- 1 tablespoon dried oregano
- ½ teaspoon celery seed
- Pinch freshly ground black pepper
- ½ cup olive oil

Directions:

1. Mix the vinegar, honey, garlic, parsley, oregano, celery seed, and pepper in a small bowl. Whisk in the olive oil until emulsified. Store the dressing in a sealed glass container in the refrigerator for up to 1 week.

Nutrition:

Calories: 100

Fat: 11g

Sodium: 1mg

Carbohydrates: 1g

Phosphorus: 1mg

Potassium: 10mg

Protein: 0g

FAJITA RUB

Preparation time: 15 minutes

Cooking time: 0 minutes

Servings: ¼ cup

Ingredients:

- 1½ teaspoons chili powder
- 1 teaspoon garlic powder
- 1 teaspoon roasted cumin seed
- 1 teaspoon dried oregano
- ½ teaspoon ground coriander
- ¼ teaspoon red pepper flakes

Directions:

1. Put the chili powder, garlic powder, cumin seed, oregano, coriander, and red pepper flakes in a blender, pulse until ground and well combined. Transfer the spice mixture and store for up to 6 months.

Nutrition:

Calories: 1

Fat: 0g

Carbohydrates: 0g

Phosphorus: 2mg

Potassium: 7mg

Sodium: 7mg

Protein: 0g

Dried Herb Rub

Preparation time: 15 minutes

Cooking time: 0 minutes

Servings: 1/3 cup

Ingredients:

- 1 tablespoon dried thyme
- 1 tablespoon dried oregano
- 1 tablespoon dried parsley
- 2 teaspoons dried basil
- 2 teaspoons ground coriander
- 2 teaspoons onion powder
- 1 teaspoon ground cumin
- 1 teaspoon garlic powder
- 1 teaspoon paprika
- ½ teaspoon cayenne pepper

Directions:

1. Put the thyme, oregano, parsley, basil, coriander, onion powder, cumin, garlic powder, paprika, and cayenne pepper in a blender, and pulse until the ingredients are ground and well combined. Transfer the rub to a small container with a lid. Store in a cool, dry area for up to 6 months.

Nutrition:

Calories: 3

Fat: 0g

Carbohydrates: 1g

Phosphorus: 3mg

Potassium: 16mg

Sodium: 1mg

Protein: 0g

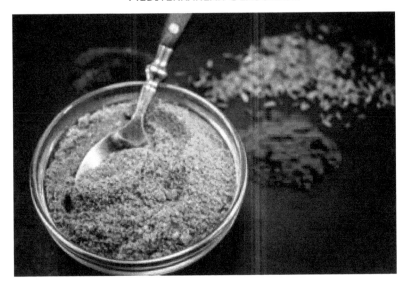

Preparation time: 15 minutes

Cooking time: 0 minutes

Servings: 1

Ingredients:

- 2 tablespoons dried oregano
- 1 tablespoon dried thyme
- 2 teaspoons dried rosemary, chopped finely or crushed
- 2 teaspoons dried basil
- 1 teaspoon dried marjoram
  1 teaspoon dried parsley flakes

Directions:

1. Mix the oregano, thyme, rosemary, basil, marjoram, and parsley in a small bowl until well combined. Transfer then store.

Nutrition:

Calories: 1

Fat: 0g

Carbohydrates: 0g

Phosphorus: 1mg

Potassium: 6mg

Sodium: 0mg

Protein: 0g

HOT CURRY POWDER

Preparation time: 15 minutes

Cooking time: 0 minutes

Servings: 1 ¼ cup

Ingredients:

- ¼ cup ground cumin
- ¼ cup ground coriander
- 3 tablespoons turmeric
- 2 tablespoons sweet paprika
- 2 tablespoons ground mustard
- 1 tablespoon fennel powder
- ½ teaspoon green chili powder
- 2 teaspoons ground cardamom
- 1 teaspoon ground cinnamon
- ½ teaspoon ground cloves

Directions:

1. Pulse the cumin, coriander, turmeric, paprika, mustard, fennel powder, green chili powder, cardamom, cinnamon, plus cloves using a blender, until the fixing is ground and well combined. Transfer it to a small container, put in a cool, dry place for up to 6 months.

Nutrition:

Calories: 19

Fat: 1g

Carbohydrates: 3g

Phosphorus: 24mg

Potassium: 93mg

Sodium: 5mg

Protein: 1g

Cajun Seasoning

Preparation time: 15 minutes

Cooking time: 0 minutes

Servings: 1 ¼ cup

Ingredients:

- ½ cup sweet paprika
- ¼ cup garlic powder
- 3 tablespoons onion powder
- 3 tablespoons freshly ground black pepper
- 2 tablespoons dried oregano
- 1 tablespoon cayenne pepper
- 1 tablespoon dried thyme

Directions:

1. Pulse the paprika, garlic powder, onion powder, black pepper, oregano, cayenne pepper, and thyme in a blender until the fixing is ground and well combined.

Nutrition:

Calories: 7

Fat: 0g

Carbohydrates: 2g

Phosphorus: 8mg

Potassium: 40mg

Sodium: 1mg

Protein: 0g

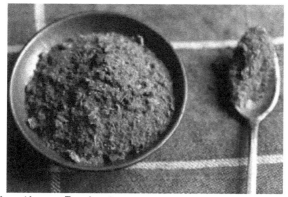

Preparation time: 5 minutes

Cooking time: 0 minutes

Servings: ½ cup

Ingredients:

- 2 teaspoons ground nutmeg
- 2 teaspoons ground coriander
- 2 teaspoons ground cumin
- 2 teaspoons turmeric
- 2 teaspoons cinnamon
- 1 teaspoon cardamom
- 1 teaspoon sweet paprika
- 1 teaspoon ground mace
- 1 teaspoon freshly ground black pepper
- 1 teaspoon cayenne pepper
- ½ teaspoon ground allspice
- ½ teaspoon ground cloves

Directions:

1. Mix the nutmeg, coriander, cumin, turmeric, cinnamon, cardamom, paprika, mace, black pepper, cayenne pepper, allspice, and cloves in a small bowl. Store.

Nutrition:

Calories: 5

Fat: 0g

Carbohydrates: 1g

Phosphorus: 3mg

Potassium: 17mg

Sodium: 1mg

Protein: 0g

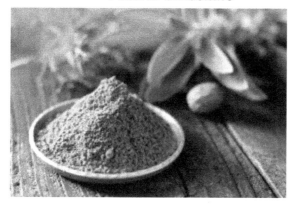

Preparation time: 15 minutes

Cooking time: 0 minutes

Servings: ½ cup

Ingredients:

- 2 tablespoons ground thyme
- 2 tablespoons ground marjoram
- 1 tablespoon ground sage
- 1 tablespoon ground celery seed
- 1 teaspoon ground rosemary
- 1 teaspoon freshly ground black pepper

Directions:

1. Mix the thyme, marjoram, sage, celery seed, rosemary, and pepper in a small bowl. Store for up to 6 months.

Nutrition:

Calories: 3

Fat: 0g

Carbohydrates: 0g

Phosphorus: 3mg

Potassium: 10mg

Sodium: 1mg

Protein: 0g

Preparation time: 15 minutes

Cooking time: 0 minutes

Servings: 1 cup

Ingredients:

- ½ cup dried thyme
- 3 tablespoons dried marjoram
- 3 tablespoons dried savory
- 2 tablespoons dried rosemary
- 2 teaspoons dried lavender flowers
- 1 teaspoon ground fennel

Directions:

1. Put the thyme, marjoram, savory, rosemary, lavender, and fennel in a blender and pulse a few times to combine. Store for up to 6 months.

Nutrition:

Calories: 3

Fat: 0g

Carbohydrates: 1g

Phosphorus: 2mg

Potassium: 9mg

Sodium: 0mg

LAMB AND PORK SEASONING

Preparation time: 15 minutes

Cooking time: 0 minutes

Servings: ½ cup

Ingredients:

- ¼ cup celery seed
- 2 tablespoons dried oregano
- 2 tablespoons onion powder
- 1 tablespoon dried thyme
- 1½ teaspoons garlic powder
- 1 teaspoon crushed bay leaf
- 1 teaspoon freshly ground black pepper
- 1 teaspoon ground allspice

Directions:

1. Pulse the celery seed, oregano, onion powder, thyme, garlic powder, bay leaf, pepper, and allspice in a blender a few times. Transfer the herb mixture to a small container; then, you can store it in a cool, dry place for up to 6 months.

Nutrition:

Calories: 8

Fat: 0g

Carbohydrates: 1g

Phosphorus: 9mg

Potassium: 29mg

Sodium: 2mg

Protein: 0g

ASIAN SEASONING

Preparation time: 5 minutes

Cooking time: 0 minutes

Servings: ½ cup

Ingredients:

- 2 tablespoons sesame seeds
- 2 tablespoons onion powder
- 2 tablespoons crushed star anise pods
- 2 tablespoons ground ginger
- 1 teaspoon ground allspice
- ½ teaspoon cardamom
- ½ teaspoon ground cloves

Directions:

1. Mix the sesame seeds, onion powder, star anise, ginger, allspice, cardamom, and cloves in a small bowl. Transfer the spice mixture to a container with a cover. Store for up to 6 months.

Nutrition:

Calories: 10

Fat: 0g

Carbohydrates: 1g

Phosphorus: 11mg

Potassium: 24mg

Sodium: 5mg

Protein: 0g

Preparation time: 15 minutes

Cooking time: 0 minutes

Servings: ½ cup

Ingredients:

- 2 tablespoons onion powder
- 1 tablespoon dry mustard
- 2 teaspoons sweet paprika
- 2 teaspoons garlic powder
- 1 teaspoon dried thyme
- ½ teaspoon celery seeds
- ½ teaspoon freshly ground black pepper

Directions:

1. Mix the onion powder, mustard, paprika, garlic powder, thyme, celery seeds, and pepper until well combined in a small bowl. Store for up to 6 months.

Nutrition:

Calories: 5

Fat: 0g

Carbohydrates: 1g

Phosphorus: 6mg

Potassium: 17mg

Sodium: 1mg

Protein: 1g

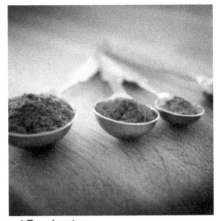

Preparation time: 15 minutes

Cooking time: 0 minutes

Servings: 2 tbsp

Ingredients:

- 1 teaspoon dried thyme leaves
- 1 teaspoon dried marjoram leaves
- 1 teaspoon dried basil leaves
- 1 teaspoon dried oregano leaves
- ½ teaspoon onion powder
- ½ teaspoon garlic powder
- ½ teaspoon ground mustard
- ¼ teaspoon freshly ground black pepper
- ¼ teaspoon paprika

Directions:

1. Combine the thyme, marjoram, basil, oregano, onion powder, garlic powder, ground mustard, pepper, and paprika. Transfer and store at room temperature for up to 6 months.

Nutrition:

Calories: 4

Fat: 0g

Sodium: 0mg

Potassium: 17mg

Phosphorus: 4mg

Carbohydrates: 1g

Protein: 0g

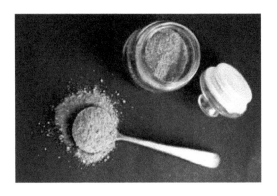

Preparation time: 15 minutes

Cooking time: 0 minutes

Servings: 3 tbsp

Ingredients:

- 1½ teaspoons turmeric
- 1½ teaspoons paprika
- 1 teaspoon ground coriander
- 1 teaspoon ground ginger
- 1 teaspoon dry mustard
- 1 teaspoon ground cumin
- 1 teaspoon dried mint leaves, crushed
- 1 teaspoon red pepper flakes

Directions:

1. Combine the turmeric, paprika, coriander, ginger, dry mustard, cumin, mint, and red pepper flakes and store for up to 6 months.

Nutrition:

Calories: 5

Fat: 0g

Sodium: 1mg

Potassium: 30mg

Phosphorus: 6mg

Carbohydrates: 1g

Protein: 0g

Tex-Mex Seasoning Mix

Preparation time: 10 minutes

Cooking time: 0 minutes

Servings: 2 tbsp

Ingredients:

- 1 tablespoon chili powder
- ½ teaspoon ground cumin
- ½ teaspoon dried oregano leaves
- ½ teaspoon garlic powder
- ½ teaspoon onion powder
- ½ teaspoon cayenne pepper
- ½ teaspoon red pepper flakes

Directions:

1. Combine the chili powder, cumin, oregano, garlic powder, onion powder, cayenne pepper, and red pepper flakes. Store for up to 6 months.

Nutrition:

Calories: 7

Fat: 0g

Sodium: 39mg

Potassium: 38mg

Phosphorus: 7mg

Carbohydrates: 1g

Protein: 0g

DUXELLES

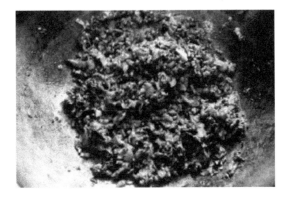

Preparation time: 15 minutes

Cooking time: 15 minutes

Servings: 8

Ingredients:

- 1 (8-ounce) package sliced cremini mushrooms
- 3 scallions, white and green parts
- 3 garlic cloves
- 1 tablespoon olive oil
- 1 tablespoon unsalted butter
- 1 teaspoon freshly squeezed lemon juice
- Pinch salt

Directions:

1. Finely chop the mushrooms, scallions, and garlic in a food processor or blender. Put the mushroom batter in the middle of a kitchen towel. Gather up the ends to create a pouch, and

squeeze the pouch over the sink to remove some of the mushrooms' liquid.

2. Heat-up olive oil and butter in a large skillet over medium-high heat. Add the drained mushroom mixture to the skillet and sprinkle with the lemon juice and salt.

3. Sauté for 8 to 12 minutes, stirring frequently, or until the mushrooms are browned. This mixture can be refrigerated up to 4 days or frozen up to 1 month.

Nutrition:

Calories: 37

Fat: 3g

Sodium: 22mg

Potassium: 141mg

Phosphorus: 37mg

Carbohydrates: 2g

Protein: 1g

Chicken Stock

Preparation time: 15 minutes

Cooking time: 25 minutes

Servings: 4

Ingredients:

- 1 tablespoon olive oil
- 1 bone-in skin-on chicken breast (3 to 4 ounces)
- Pinch salt
- 1 onion, unpeeled, sliced
- 1 carrot, unpeeled, sliced
- 1 bay leaf
- 5 cups of water

Directions:

1. Heat-up olive oil in a large saucepan over medium-high heat. Sprinkle the chicken with salt and add to the pan, skin-side down. Brown for 2 minutes.
2. Put the onion plus carrot and cook within 1 minute longer. Add the bay leaf and water and bring to a boil. Adjust the heat to medium-low and simmer within 20 to 22 minutes, stirring occasionally. Remove the scum that pops to the surface.
3. Drain or strain the stock through a fine-mesh colander into a bowl. You can reserve the chicken breast for other recipes,

although it may be tough after cooking. Discard the remaining solids.

4. Fridge the broth and skim off any fat that rises to the top. You can freeze this stock in 1-cup measures to use in recipes. Store freezer up to 3 months.

Nutrition:

Calories: 37

Fat: 2g

Sodium: 22mg

Potassium: 85mg

Phosphorus: 30mg

Carbohydrates: 2g

Protein: 3g

VEGETABLE BROTH

Preparation time: 15 minutes

Cooking time: 27 minutes

Servings: 4

Ingredients:

- 1 tablespoon olive oil
- 1 unpeeled onion, sliced
- 2 unpeeled garlic cloves, crushed
- 2 unpeeled carrots, sliced
- 2 celery stalks, cut into 2-inch pieces
- 1 bay leaf
- 1 teaspoon dried basil leaves
- 5 cups of water

Directions:

1. Heat-up olive oil in a large saucepan over medium-high heat. Sauté the onion, garlic, carrot, and celery for 5 minutes, stirring frequently or lightly browned.
2. Add the bay leaf, basil, and water to the saucepan and bring to a boil. Adjust the heat to medium-low, then simmer for 20 to 22 minutes, stirring occasionally. Skim off and discard any scum that rises to the surface.

3. Strain the stock to a fine-mesh colander into a bowl. Discard the solids. Fridge the broth and remove any fat that rises to the top. You can freeze this broth in 1-cup measures to use in recipes.

Nutrition:

Calories: 31

Fat: 2g

Sodium: 21mg

Potassium: 110mg

Phosphorus: 14mg

Carbohydrates: 4g

Protein: 0g

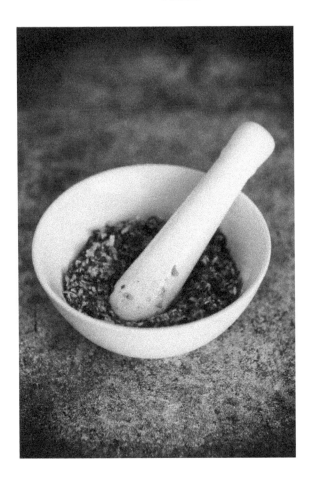

Preparation time: 15 minutes

Cooking time: 0 minutes

Servings: 16

Ingredients:

- 2 cups fresh basil leaves
- ½ cup flat-leaf parsley
- 2 garlic cloves, sliced
- 3 tablespoons olive oil, + more for drizzling
- 2 tablespoons grated Parmesan cheese
- 2 tablespoons chopped walnuts
- 2 tablespoons water
- 1 tablespoon freshly squeezed lemon juice

Directions:

1. Process the basil, parsley, garlic, olive oil, cheese, walnuts, water, and lemon juice in a blender or food processor. Put the pesto in a bowl and drizzle more olive oil on top to prevent browning. Store.

Nutrition:

Calories: 34

Fat: 3g

Sodium: 16mg

Potassium: 35mg

Phosphorus: 13mg

Carbohydrates: 1g

Protein: 1g

RANCH SEASONING MIX

Preparation time: 15 minutes

Cooking time: 0 minutes

Servings: 1/3 cup

Ingredients:

- 2 tablespoons dried buttermilk powder
- 1 tablespoon cornstarch
- 1 tablespoon dried parsley
- 1 teaspoon dried dill weed
- 1 teaspoon dried chives
- ½ teaspoon garlic powder
- ½ teaspoon onion powder
- ¼ teaspoon freshly ground black pepper

Directions:

1. Combine the buttermilk powder, cornstarch, parsley, dill weed, chives, garlic powder, onion powder, and pepper and keep in a small jar with a tight lid at room temperature for up to 6 months.

Nutrition:

Calories: 8

Fat: >1g

Sodium: 1mg

Potassium: 27mg

Phosphorus: 4mg

Carbohydrates: 1g

Protein: >1g

POULTRY SEASONING MIX

Preparation time: 15 minutes

Cooking time: 0 minutes

Servings: 2 tbsp

Ingredients:

- 2 teaspoons dried thyme leaves
- 2 teaspoons dried basil leaves
- 1½ teaspoons dried marjoram leaves
- ¼ teaspoon onion powder
- ¼ teaspoon garlic powder
- 1/8 teaspoon freshly ground black pepper

Directions:

1. Combine the thyme, basil, marjoram, onion powder, garlic powder, and pepper in a small bowl and mix. Store at room temperature. You can grind all of these ingredients together to make a more like commercial poultry seasoning.

Nutrition:

Calories: 21

Fat: >1g

Sodium: 23mg

Potassium: 132mg

Phosphorus: 17mg

Carbohydrates: 5g

Protein: 1g

HOMEMADE MUSTARD

Preparation time: 15 minutes

Cooking time: 0 minutes

Servings: ½ cup

Ingredients:

- ¼ cup dry mustard
- 3 tablespoons mustard seeds
- 3 tablespoons apple cider vinegar
- 3 tablespoons water
- 2 tablespoons freshly squeezed lemon juice
- ½ teaspoon turmeric

Directions:

1. Combine the dry mustard, mustard seeds, vinegar, water, lemon juice, and turmeric in a jar with a tight-fitting lid and stir to combine.
2. Refrigerate the mustard for 3 days, stirring once a day and adding a bit more water every day if necessary.
3. After three days, the mustard is ready to use. You can process the mixture in a food processor or blender if you'd like smoother mustard. Refrigerate up to 2 weeks.

Nutrition:

Calories: 9

Fat: 0g

Sodium: 0mg

Potassium: 16mg

Phosphorus: 13mg

Carbohydrates: 1g

Protein: 0g

CRANBERRY KETCHUP

Preparation time: 15 minutes

Cooking time: 20 minutes

Servings: 1 cup

Ingredients:

- 2 cups fresh cranberries
- 1 1/3 cups water
- 3 tablespoons brown sugar
- Juice of 1 lemon
- 2 teaspoons yellow mustard
- ¼ teaspoon onion powder
- Pinch salt
- Pinch ground cloves

Directions:

1. Stir together the cranberries, water, brown sugar, lemon juice, mustard, onion powder, salt, and cloves in a medium saucepan on medium heat, then boil.
2. Reduce the heat to low and simmer until the cranberries have popped, about 15 minutes. Mash using an immersion blender the ingredients right in the saucepan.
3. After mashing, simmer the ketchup for another 5 minutes until thickened. Let the ketchup cool for 1 hour in the saucepan, then put it into an airtight container and store.

Nutrition:

Calories: 13

Fat: 0g

Sodium: 19mg

Potassium: 17mg

Phosphorus: 3mg

Carbohydrates: 3g

Protein: 0g

GRAINY MUSTARD

Preparation time: 15 minutes

Cooking time: 0 minutes

Servings: ½ cup

Ingredients:

- ¼ cup dry mustard
- ¼ cup mustard seeds
- ¼ cup apple cider vinegar
- 3 tablespoons water
- 2 tablespoons freshly squeezed lemon juice
- ½ teaspoon ground turmeric
- 1/8 teaspoon salt

Directions:

1. Mix the mustard, mustard seeds, vinegar, water, lemon juice, turmeric, and salt in a jar with a tight-fitting lid.
2. Refrigerate the mustard for 5 days, stirring once a day and adding a bit more water every day, as the mustard will thicken as it stands. After 5 days, the mustard is ready to use. Fridge for up to 2 weeks.

Nutrition:

Calories: 22

Fat: 2g

Sodium: 13mg

Phosphorus: 9mg

Potassium: 13mg

Carbohydrates: 1g

Protein: 1g

Salsa Verde

Preparation time: 20 minutes

Cooking time: 15 minutes

Servings: 2 cups

Ingredients:

- 2 cups halved tomatillos or 1 can tomatillos, drained
- 3 scallions, chopped
- 1 jalapeño pepper, chopped
- 2 tablespoons extra-virgin olive oil
- 1/3 cup cilantro leaves
- 2 tablespoons freshly squeezed lime juice
- 1/8 teaspoon salt

Directions:

1. Preheat the oven to 400°F. Mix the tomatillos, scallions, and jalapeño pepper on a rimmed baking sheet.
2. Drizzle using the olive oil, then toss to coat. Roast the vegetables for 12 to 17 minutes or until the tomatillos are soft and light golden brown around the edges.
3. Blend the roasted vegetables with the cilantro, lime juice, and salt in a blender or food processor. Blend until smooth. Store.

Nutrition:

Calories: 22

Fat: 2g

Sodium: 20mg

Phosphorus: 8mg

Potassium: 55mg

Carbohydrates: 1g

GRAPE SALSA

Preparation time: 15 minutes

Cooking time: 0 minutes

Servings: 2 cups

Ingredients:

- 1 cup coarsely chopped red grapes
- 1 cup coarsely chopped green grapes
- ½ cup chopped red onion
- 2 tablespoons freshly squeezed lime juice
- 1 tablespoon honey
- 1/8 teaspoon salt
- ¼ teaspoon freshly ground black pepper

Directions:

1. Mix the grapes, onion, lime juice, honey, salt, and pepper in a medium bowl. Chill within 1 to 2 hours before serving or serve immediately.

Nutrition:

Calories: 51

Fat: 0g

Sodium: 53mg

Phosphorus: 14mg

Potassium: 121mg

Carbohydrates: 14g

Protein: 1g

Apple and Brown Sugar Chutney

Preparation time: 15 minutes

Cooking time: 60 minutes

Servings: 2 cups

Ingredients:

- 3 Granny Smith apples, peeled and chopped
- 1 onion, chopped
- 1 cup of water
- ½ cup golden raisins
- 1/3 cup brown sugar
- 2 teaspoons curry powder
- 1/8 teaspoon salt
- 1/8 teaspoon freshly ground black pepper

Directions:

1. In a medium saucepan, combine the apples, onion, water, raisins, brown sugar, curry powder, salt, plus pepper, then boil over medium-high heat.
2. Adjust the heat to low, then simmer, occasionally stirring, for 45 to 55 minutes. Cool, then decant into jars or containers. Store.

Nutrition:

Calories: 27

Fat: 0g

Sodium: 11mg

Phosphorus: 6mg

Potassium: 48mg

Carbohydrates: 7g

CLASSIC SPICE BLEND

Preparation time: 10 minutes

Cooking time: 0 minutes

Servings: 2 tbsp

Ingredients:

- 1 tablespoon whole black peppercorns
- 2 teaspoons caraway seeds
- 2 teaspoons celery seeds
- 1 teaspoon dill seeds
- 1 teaspoon cumin seeds

Directions:

1. Grind the peppercorns, caraway seeds, celery seeds, dill seeds, and cumin in a spice blender or a mortar and pestle. Grind until the seeds are broken down, and the mixture almost becomes a powder.

Nutrition:

Calories: 2

Fat: 0g

Sodium: 0mg

Phosphorus: 3mg

Potassium: 8mg

Carbohydrates: 0g

Protein: 0g

Garlicky Sauce

Preparation time: 15 minutes

Cooking time: 0 minutes

Servings: 1

Ingredients:

- 6 tsp of lemon juice
- .25 tsp salt
- 1 head garlic
- 8 oz of olive oil

Directions:

1. Peel apart the cloves of garlic and clean them. Place the garlic, half a tablespoon of lemon juice, and salt in the bottom of a blender. Pour the olive oil slowly in a thin stream while blending.
2. The mixture should become thick and white, resembling salad dressing. Add the remaining lemon juice and continue to blend. Keeps in a container for fourteen days.

Nutrition:

Calories 103

Phosphorus 3 mg

Protein 0 g

Carbohydrates 1 g

Sodium 30 mg

Potassium 11 mg

Fat 11 g

CPSIA information can be obtained
at www.ICGtesting.com
Printed in the USA
BVHW092150220221
600778BV00008B/896

9 781801 768344